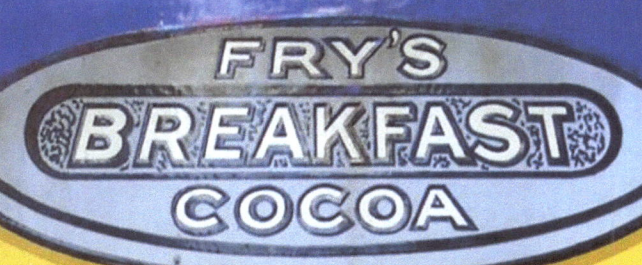

I0511356

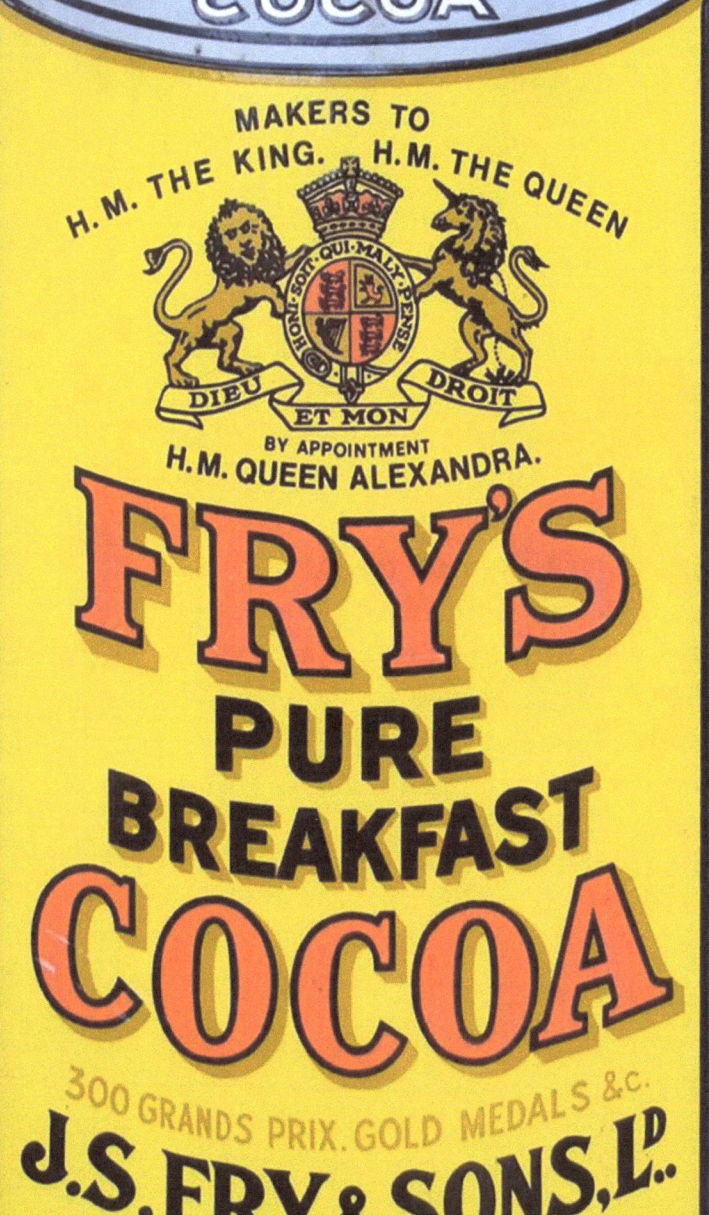

FRY'S
PURE
BREAKFAST
COCOA

MAKERS TO
H.M. THE KING. H.M. THE QUEEN
BY APPOINTMENT
H.M. QUEEN ALEXANDRA.

300 GRANDS PRIX. GOLD MEDALS &c.
J.S. FRY & SONS, Lᵈ.
BRISTOL & LONDON   REGᵈ

4 ½ D.   PER ¼ lb TIN   4 ½ D.

Discussing this image together can encourage memory recall. Give it a try.

Do you remember who taught you how to shave for the first time?

Long before Fry's chocolate was bought by Cadbury ,it was a family business started by Quaker Joseph Fry. The first factory was in Union Street in Bristol. Production on Fry's chocolate products continued there from 1777 until 1923. Under Egbert Cadbury's guidance Fry's chocolate was moved to Somerdale factory, Keynsham in Somerset. Famous Fry's products include the Fry's Cream, the milk chocolate Five Boys bar and the Fry's Turkish Delight.

.

# Let Your Beauty be Seen...

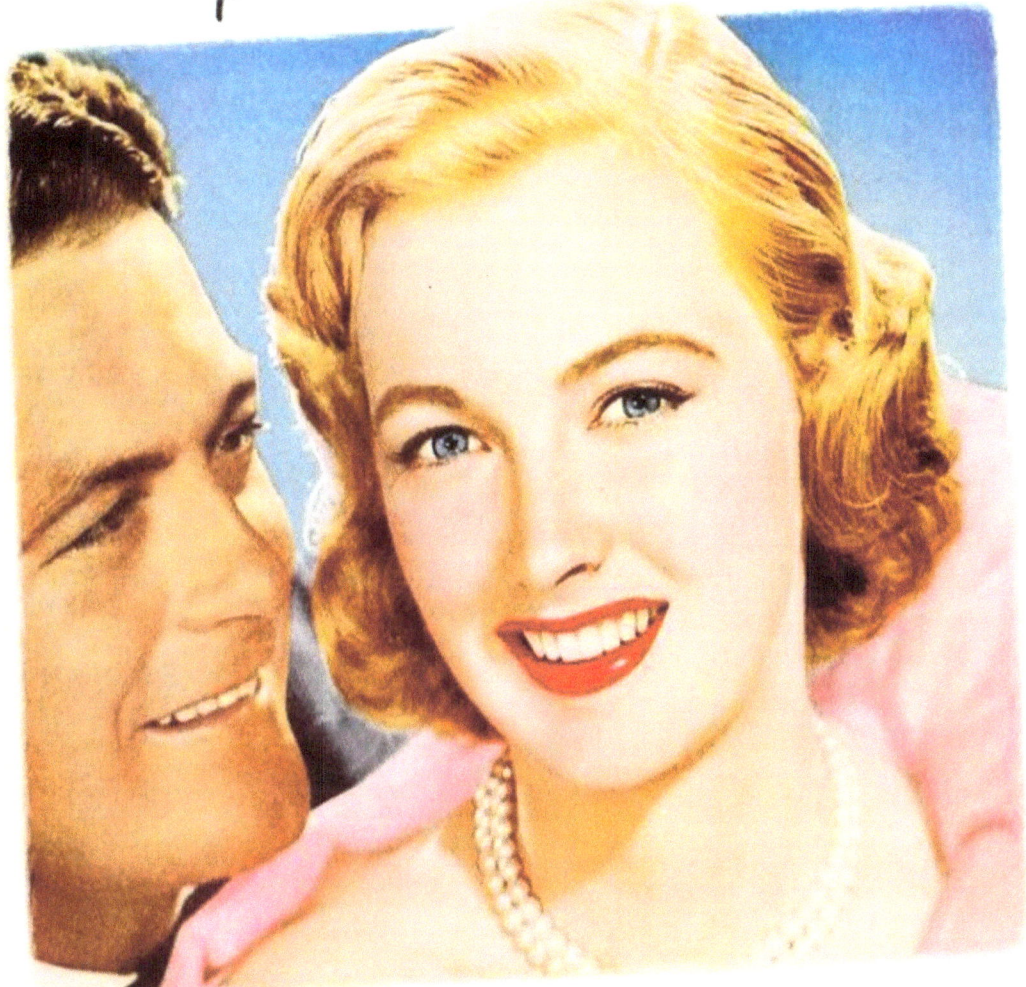

# Palmolive Brings Out Beauty

## WHILE IT CLEANS YOUR SKIN!

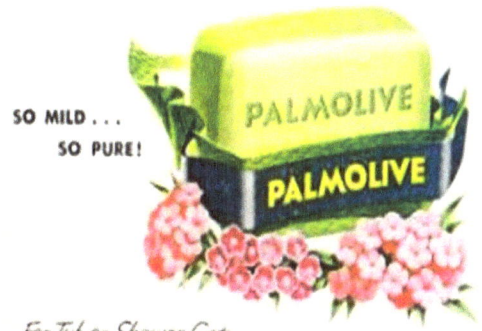

**SO MILD...
SO PURE!**

*For Tub or Shower Get
Big Bath Size Palmolive!*

**36 LEADING SKIN SPECIALISTS IN 1285
SCIENTIFIC TESTS PROVED THAT PALMOLIVE'S
BEAUTY PLAN BRINGS MOST WOMEN LOVELIER
COMPLEXIONS IN 14 DAYS**

Start Palmolive's Beauty Plan today! Discover for yourself—as women everywhere have discovered—that
Palmolive's Beauty Plan brings exciting complexion
loveliness.

Here's all you do: Gently massage Palmolive's extra-
mild, pure lather onto your skin for just a minute,
three times a day. Then rinse and pat dry. You'll see
Palmolive bring out your beauty while it cleans your skin.

*Doctors Prove Palmolive's Beauty Results!*

adflip.com

Discussing this image together can encourage memory recall. Give it a try.

Do you remember seeing Palmolive at home when you were growing up?

Palmolive is a part of the Colgate family business. William Colgate & Company originally started as a soap and candle factory long before they started producing tooth paste. The company was one of the first to sponsor soap operas in the early days of television. Do you remember any Palmolive-Colgate sponsored TV programs?

This image can be removed and used as part of our morning mnemonic routine.

.

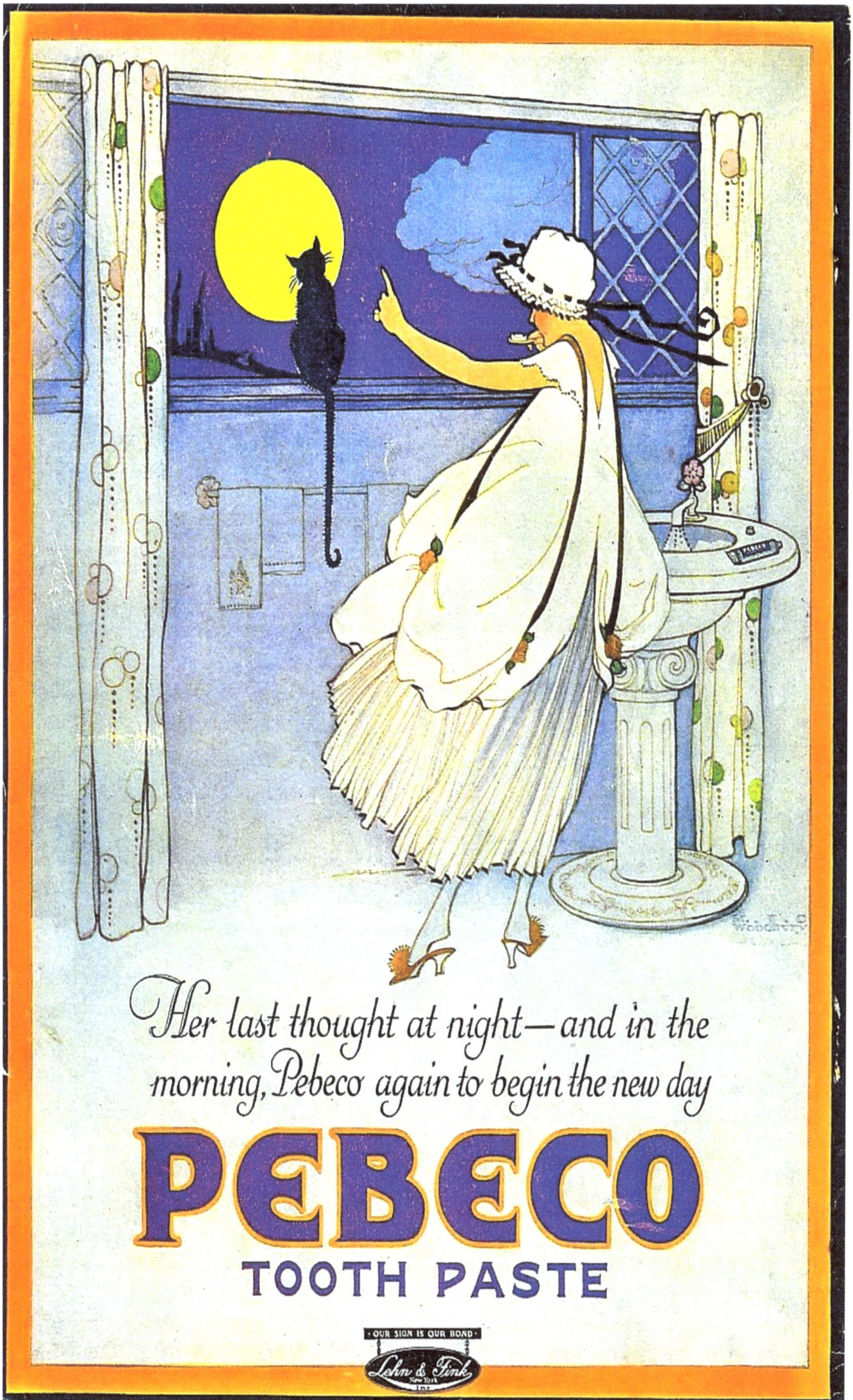

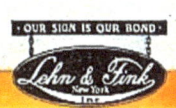

Her last thought at night—and in the morning, Pebeco again to begin the new day
PEBECO
TOOTH PASTE
· OUR SIGN IS OUR BOND ·
Lehn & Fink
New York
Inc.

Discussing this image together can encourage memory recall. Give it a try.

Did you ever get told off by your parents for not brushing your teeth as child?

Pebecco toothpaste was originally manufactured by the Beiersdorf compnay in Hamburg. It was one of the first commercial toothpastes to be mass produced.

This image can be removed and used as part of our morning mnemonic routine.

.

# McCALL'S MAGAZINE

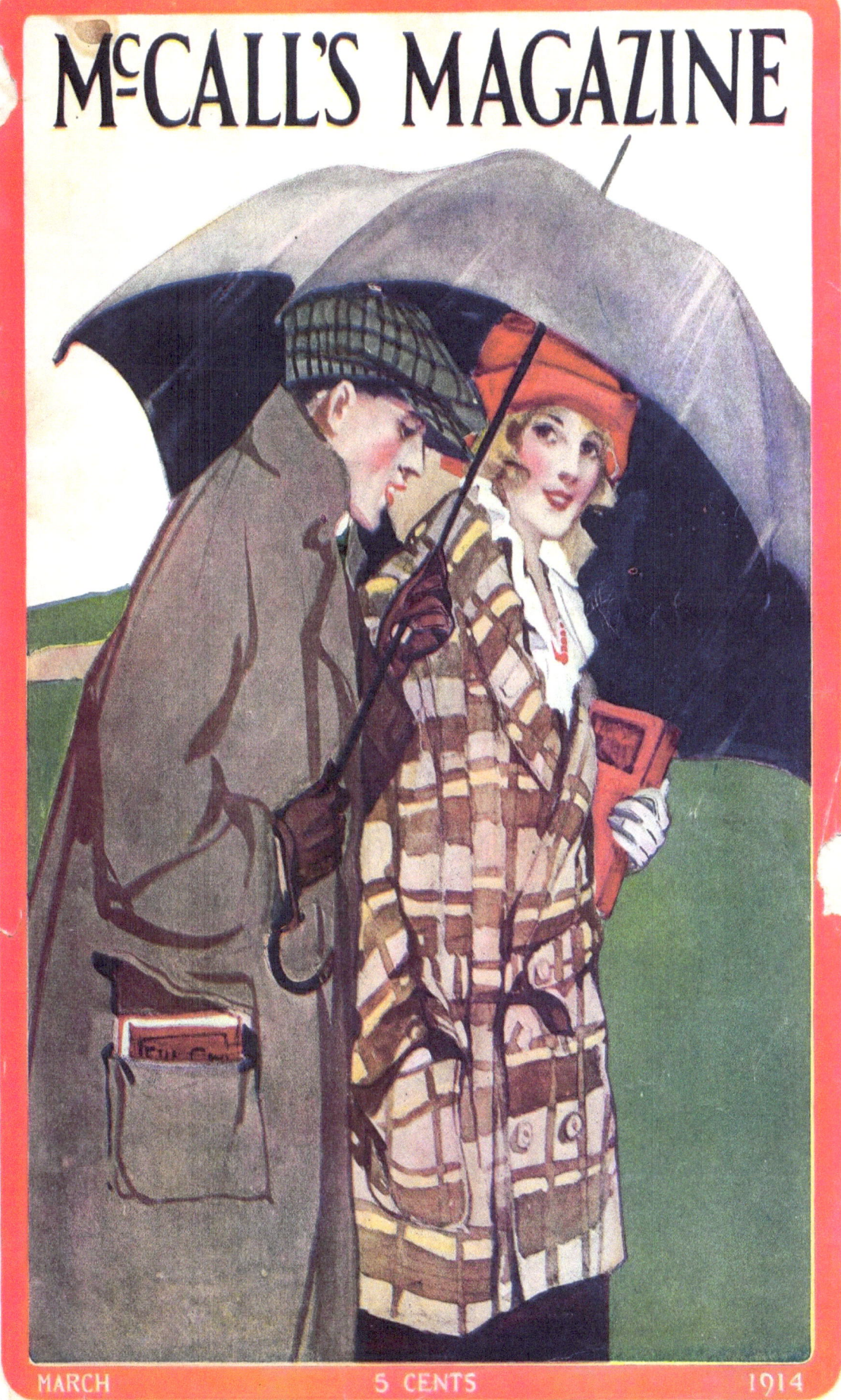

MARCH       5 CENTS       1914

Discussing this image together can encourage memory recall. Give it a try.

What was the first really expensive piece of clothing you bought with your own money?

McCall's magazine was a monthly publication. It was first published in America by Scottish immigrant James McCall to promote his own line of sewing patterns. As it grew in popularity, it expanded it's range of topics significantly. Former first lady Eleanor Rossevelt wrote a regular column from 1949 up until her death in November 1962.

This image can be removed and used as part of our morning mnemonic routine.

.

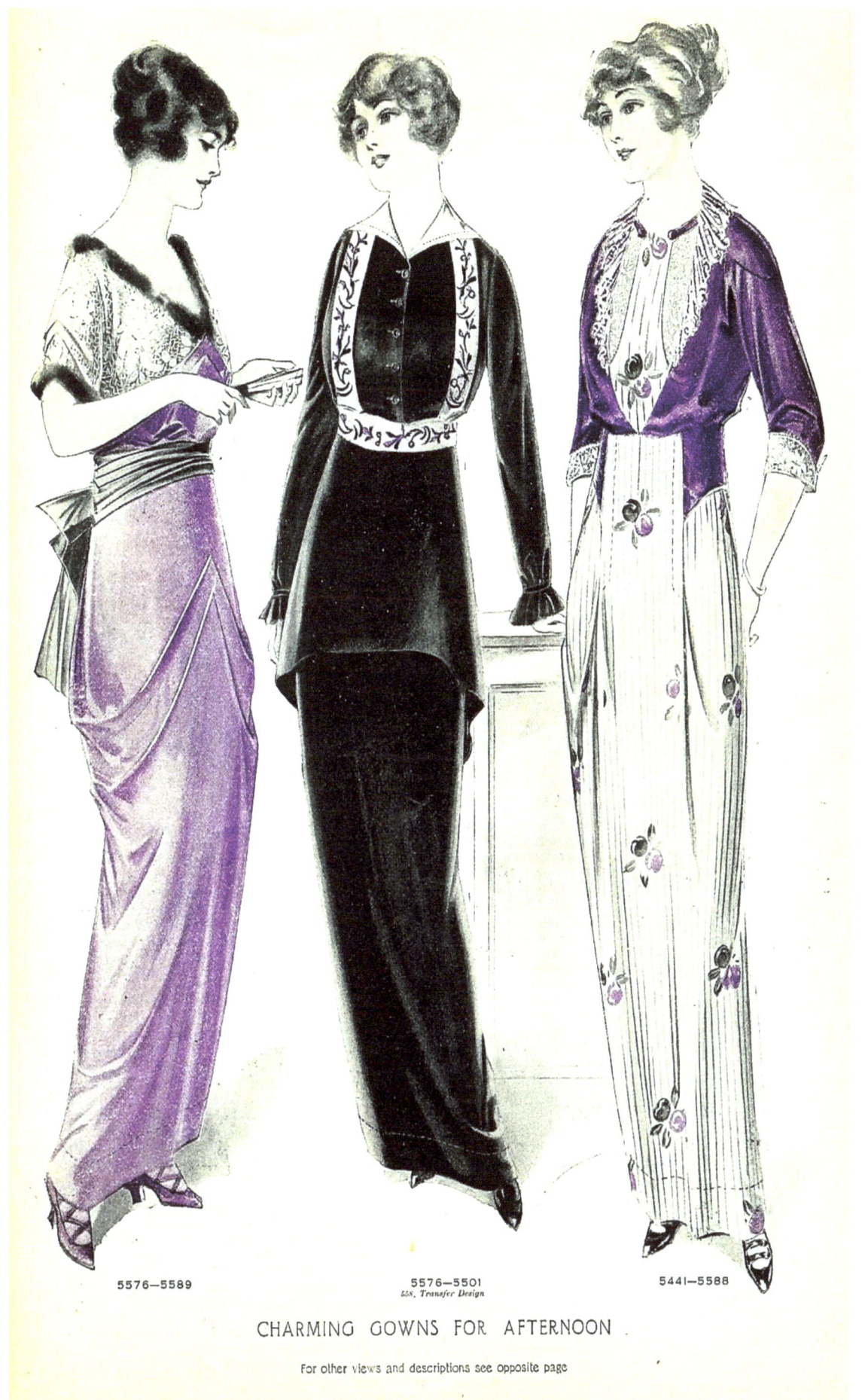

5576—5589          5576—5501          5441—5588
                   558. Transfer Design

## CHARMING GOWNS FOR AFTERNOON

For other views and descriptions see opposite page

Discussing this image together can encourage memory recall. Give it a try.

Do you remember the first expensive evening dress you bought?

Where did you buy it?

How much did it cost?

Do you remember the first suit you ever paid for yourself?

What colour was it?

This image can be removed and used as part of our morning mnemonic routine.

Discussing this image together can encourage memory recall. Give it a try.

Do you remember a time when someone else bought you a pretty dress?

Who bought it for you?

Did your parents make you where your Sunday best every weekend?

This image can be removed and used as part of our morning mnemonic routine.

.

# FRUIT.

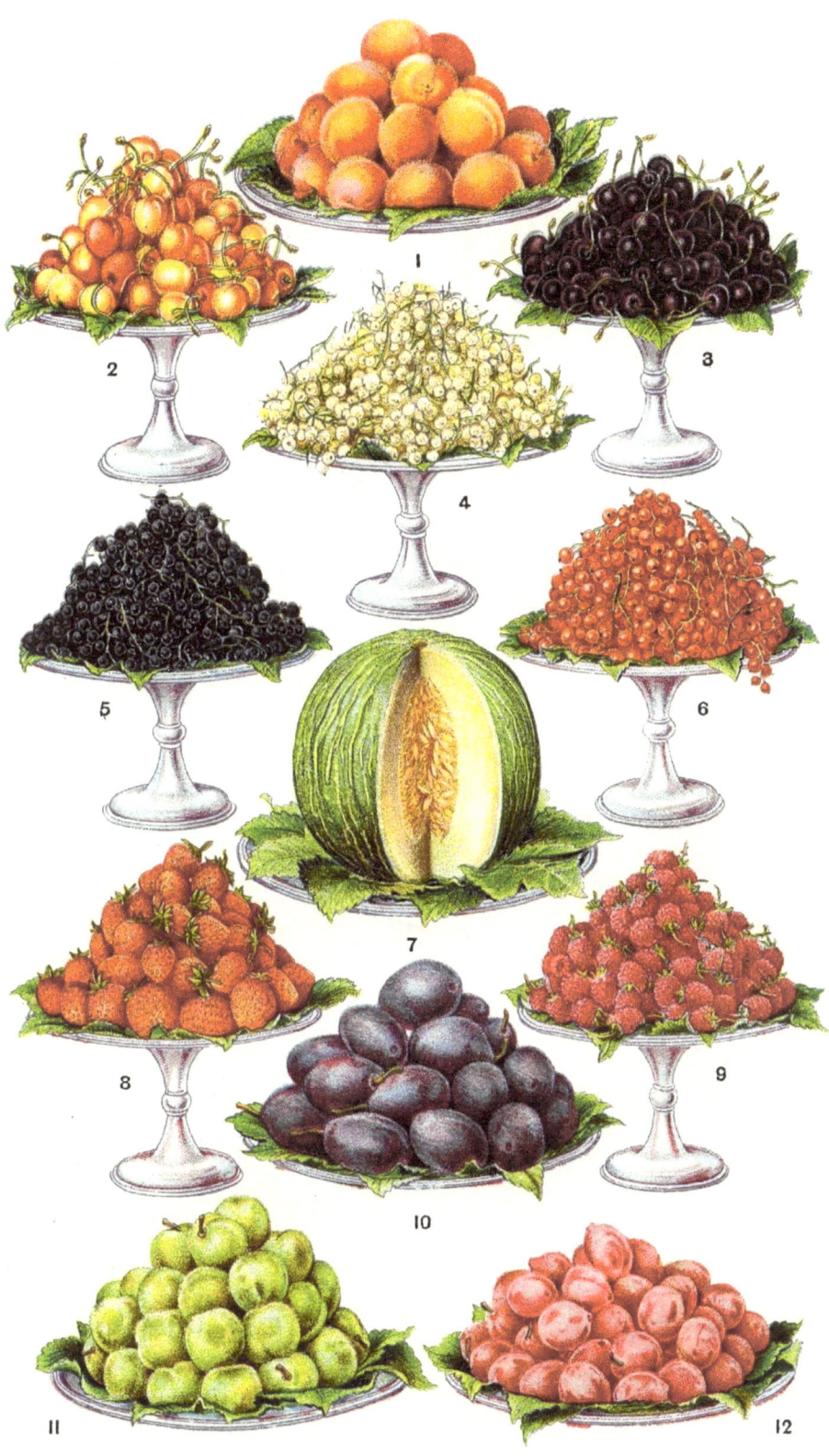

1.—Apricots.    2.—White Cherries.    3.—Black Cherries.    4.—White Currants.
5.—Black Currants.  6.—Red Currants.  7.—Melon.  8.—Strawberries.  9.—Raspberries.
10.—Plums (Black Diamonds).  11.—Greengages.  12.—Victoria Plums.

Discussing this image together can encourage memory recall. Give it a try.

Many fruits were rationed during the war. Was there any one fruit in particular you got as a treat?

An apple a day keeps the doctor away. Do you remember anyone telling you this growing up?

One Kiwi can provide you with your recommended daily intake of Vitamin C and counts as one of your five-a-day.

Bananas are delicious and nutritious. But did you know that if you freeze them, they can make a great substitute to ice-cream.

This image can be removed and used as part of our morning mnemonic routine.

.

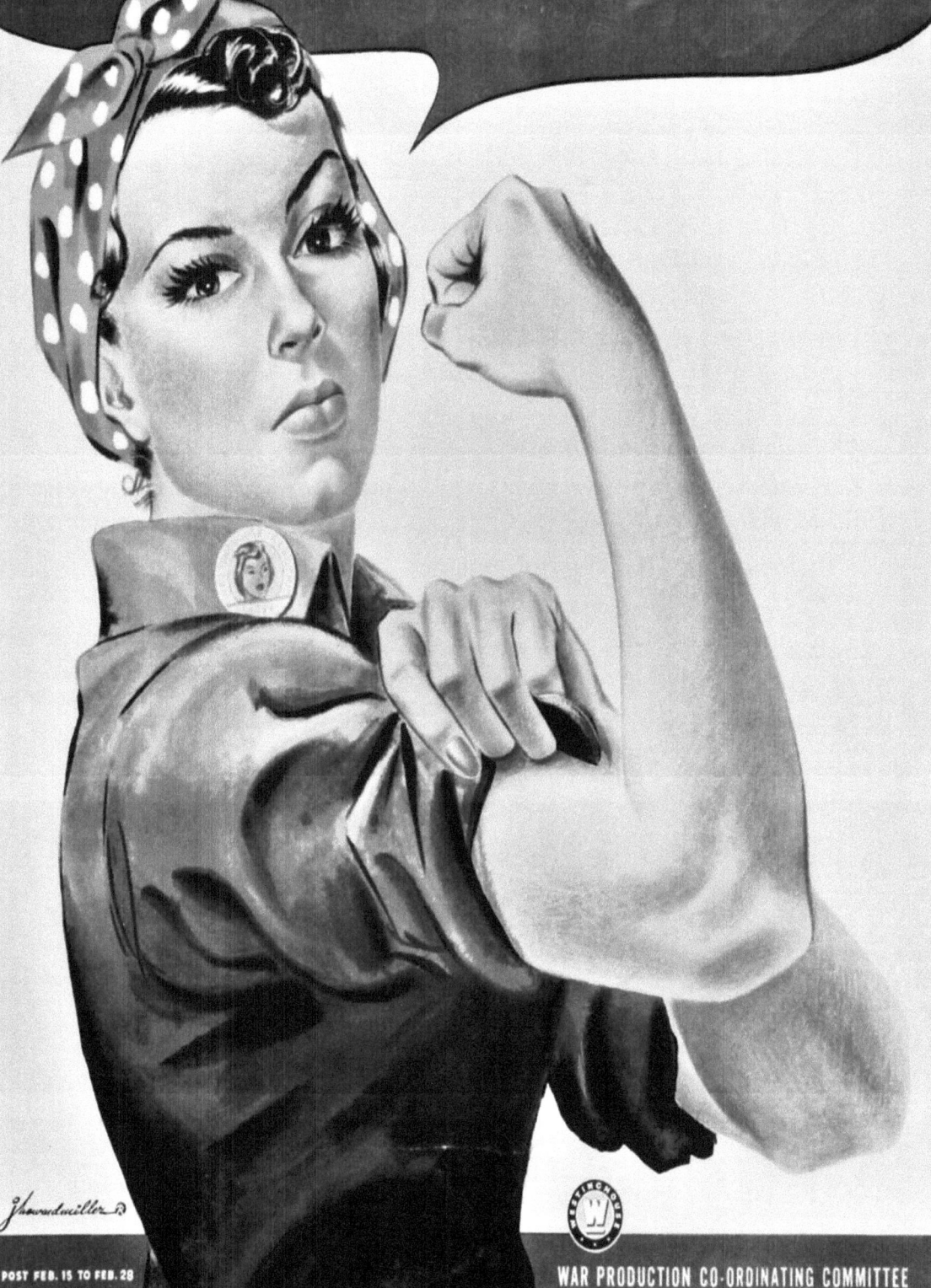

Discussing this image together can encourage memory recall. Give it a try.

Did anyone in your family leave to fight in the war?

Did anyone you know volunteer at home to help the war effort?

The iconic "We Can Do It" image was as part of the wartime propaganda in 1943. It was actually rarely seen during the war but became very popular after. The image is based on a photograph taken of a factory worker in Michigan named Geraldine Hoff.

.

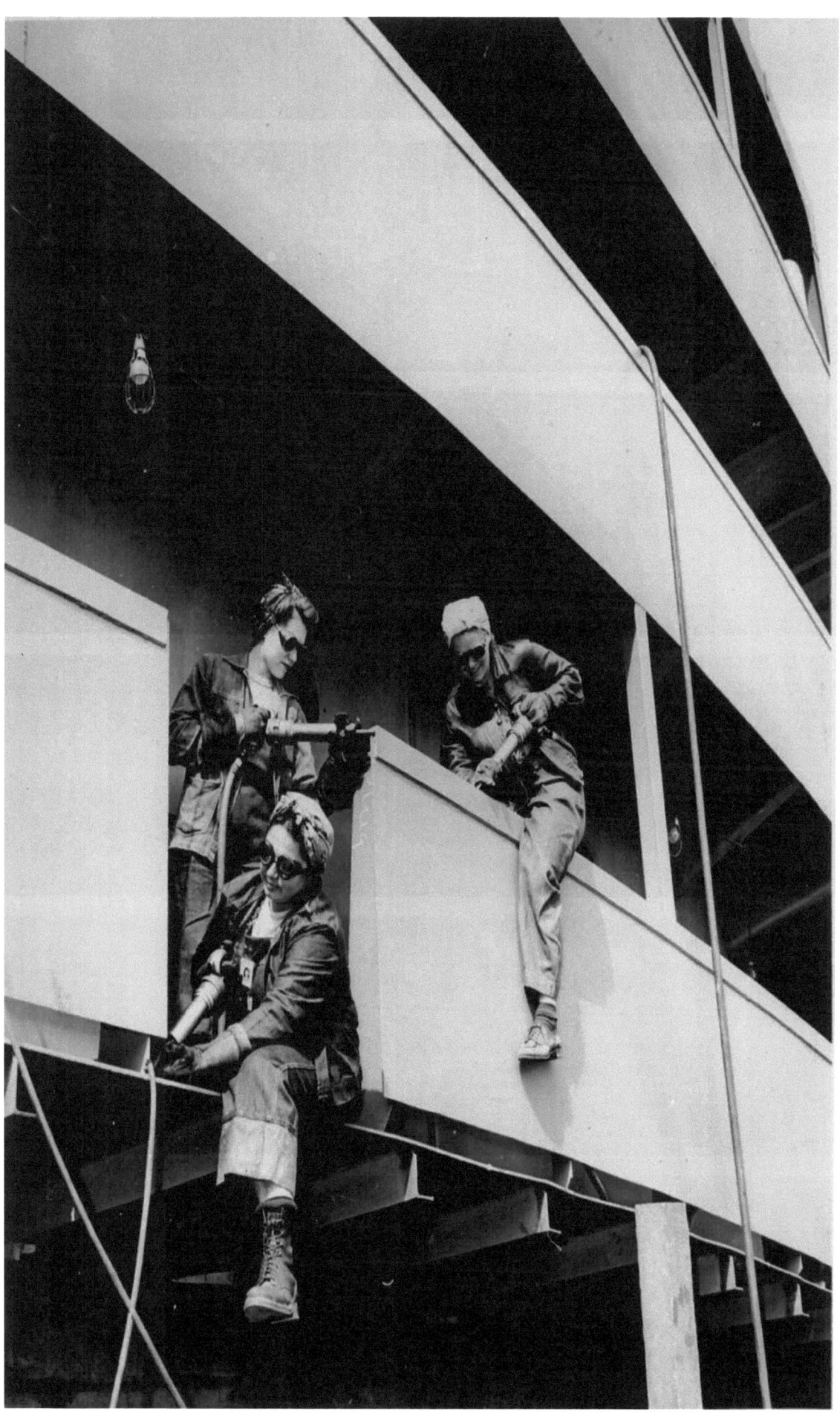

Discussing this image together can encourage memory recall. Give it a try.

Did anyone in your family leave to fight in the war?

Did anyone you know volunteer at home to help the war effort?

The iconic "We Can Do It" image was as part of the wartime propaganda in 1943. It was actually rarely seen during the war but became very popular after. The image is based on a photograph taken of a factory worker in Michigan named Geraldine Hoff.

.

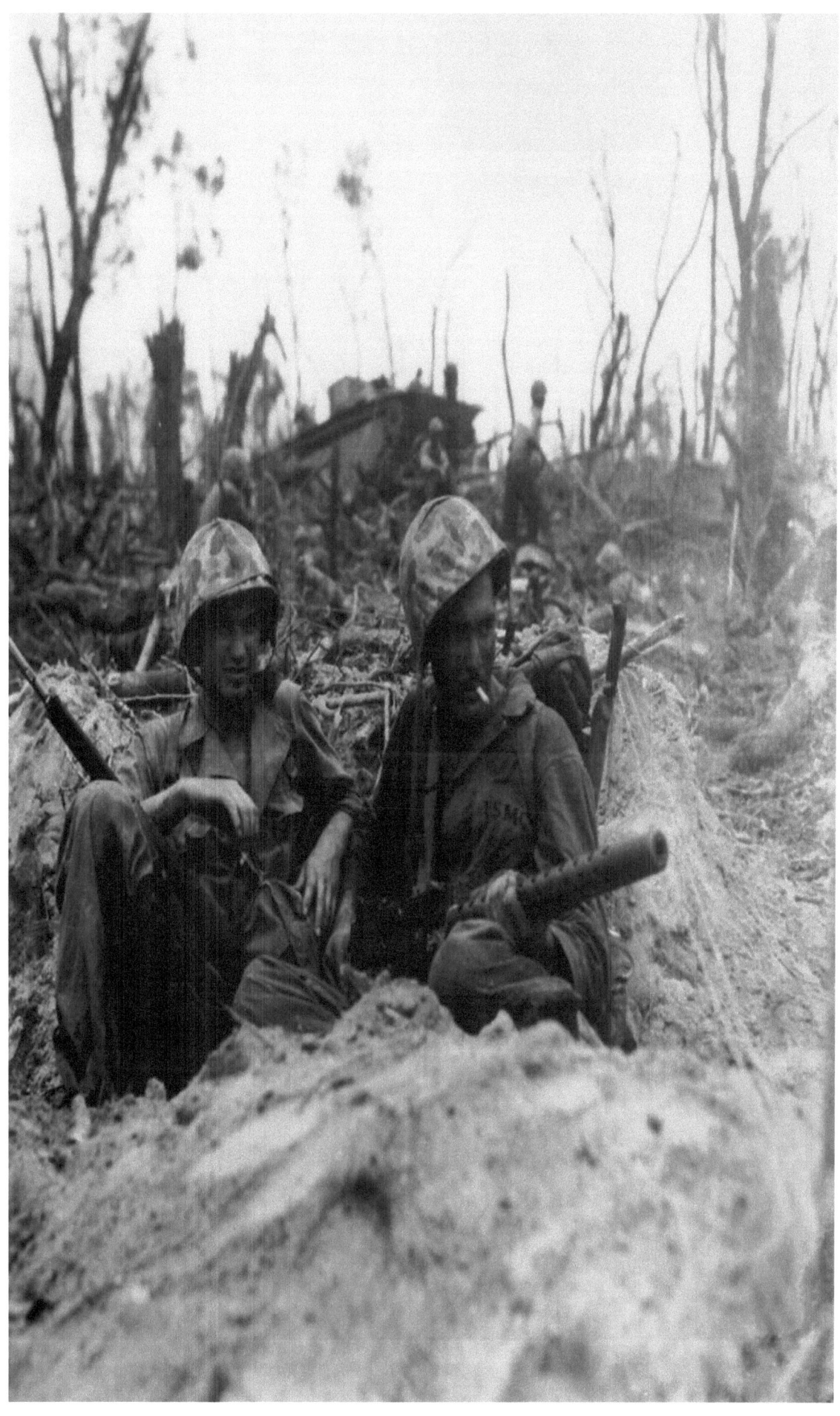

Discussing this image together can encourage memory recall. Give it a try.

Does anything specific come to mind when you think of the war?

What was it like to grow up in a wartime?

Do you remember meeting any American GIs?

In 1942 many British soldiers were away fightoing the war, the American GIs were preparing for assault. To improve moral, the GIs were invited to spend Christmas with British families. The GIs were given extra rations including Coca Cola and nylon stockings as gifts for the British hospitality.

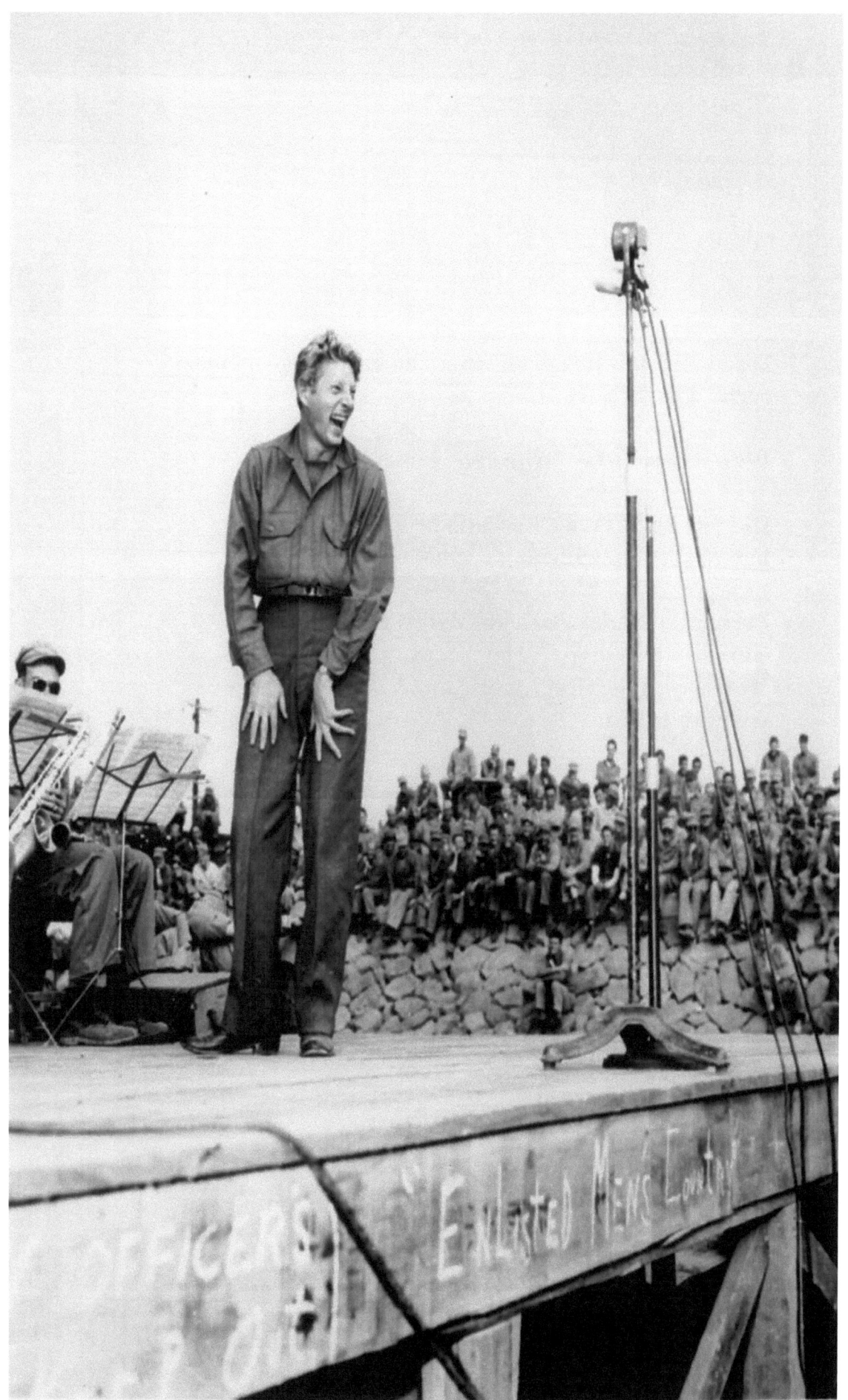

Discussing this image together can encourage memory recall. Give it a try.

Who was your favourite entertainer growing up?

Did you have favourite radio or TV show that you had to keep up with?

Performer Danny Kaye toured with the USO to entertain and support the troops during the war. He was also the first American performer to visit postwar Tokyo.

.

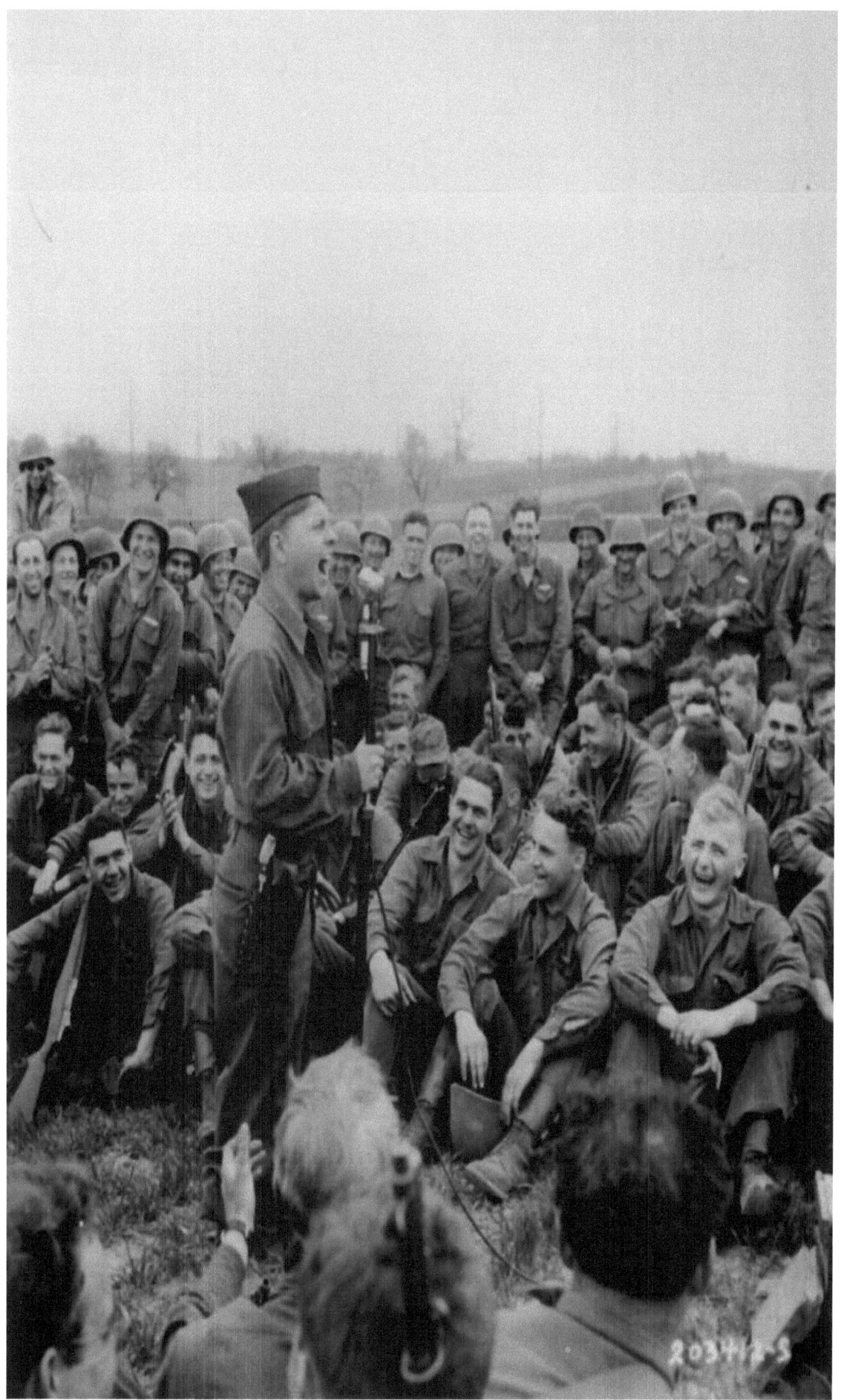

Discussing this image together can encourage memory recall. Give it a try.

Did you have a favourite actor from radio, TV or movies when you were growing up?

Do you remember the first record you bought with your own money?

Who was your favourite singer?

Mickey Rooney was the top box office draw of 1939. He starred as the character Andy Hardy in 15 films from the 1930s through to the 1940s. He was drafted to entertain the troops during the war. He earned a bronze star for performing in combat zones.

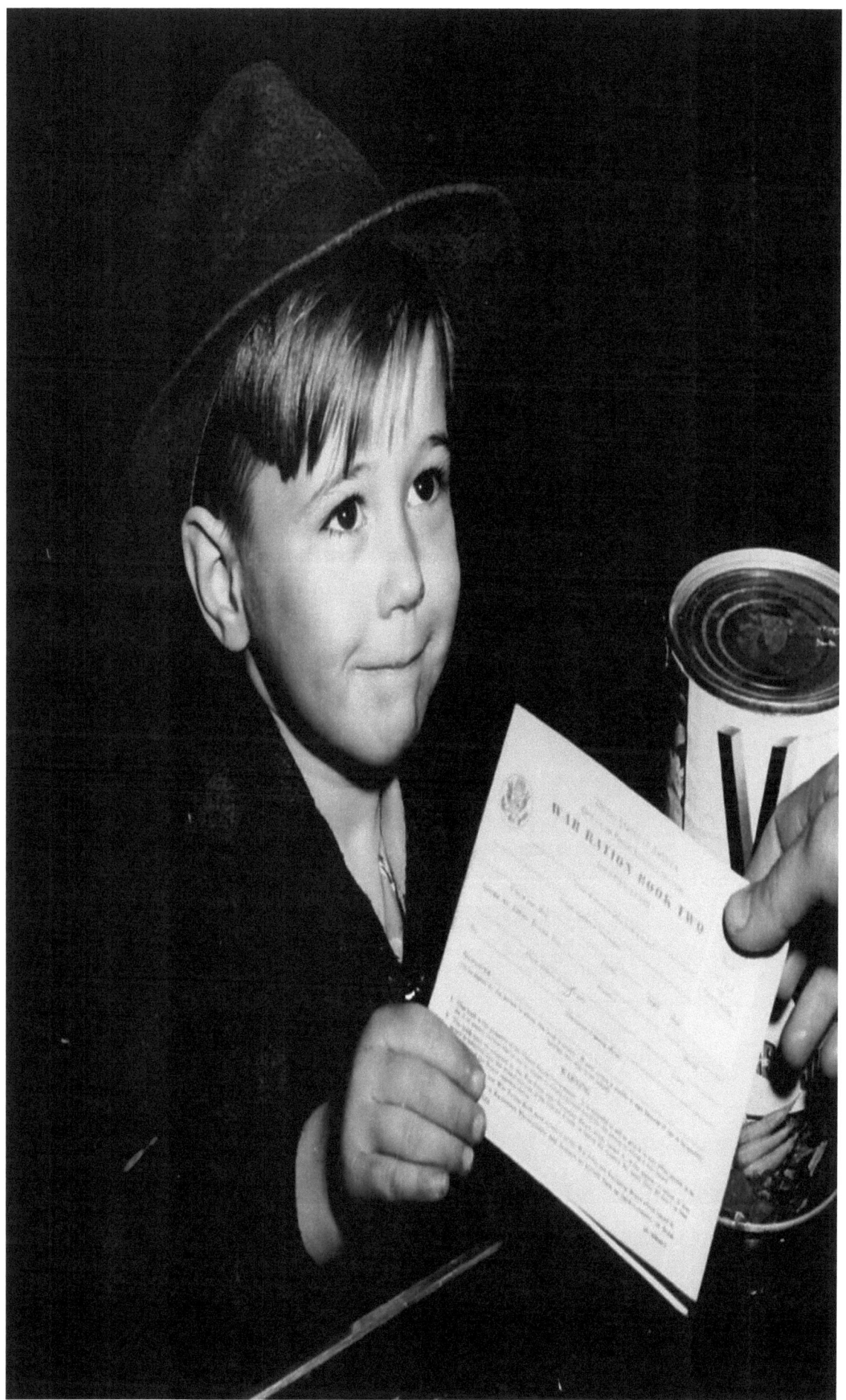

Discussing this image together can encourage memory recall. Give it a try.

Do you remember having a ration book?

Which shop did your family get its rations from?

What did you miss most during the rationing?

Do you remember when rationing came to an end after the war?

During the war some fruits and vegetables became almost unobtainable. Items such as lemons and bananas were not available for the most part of the war. White bread was also strictly rationed and replaced by wholemead bread.

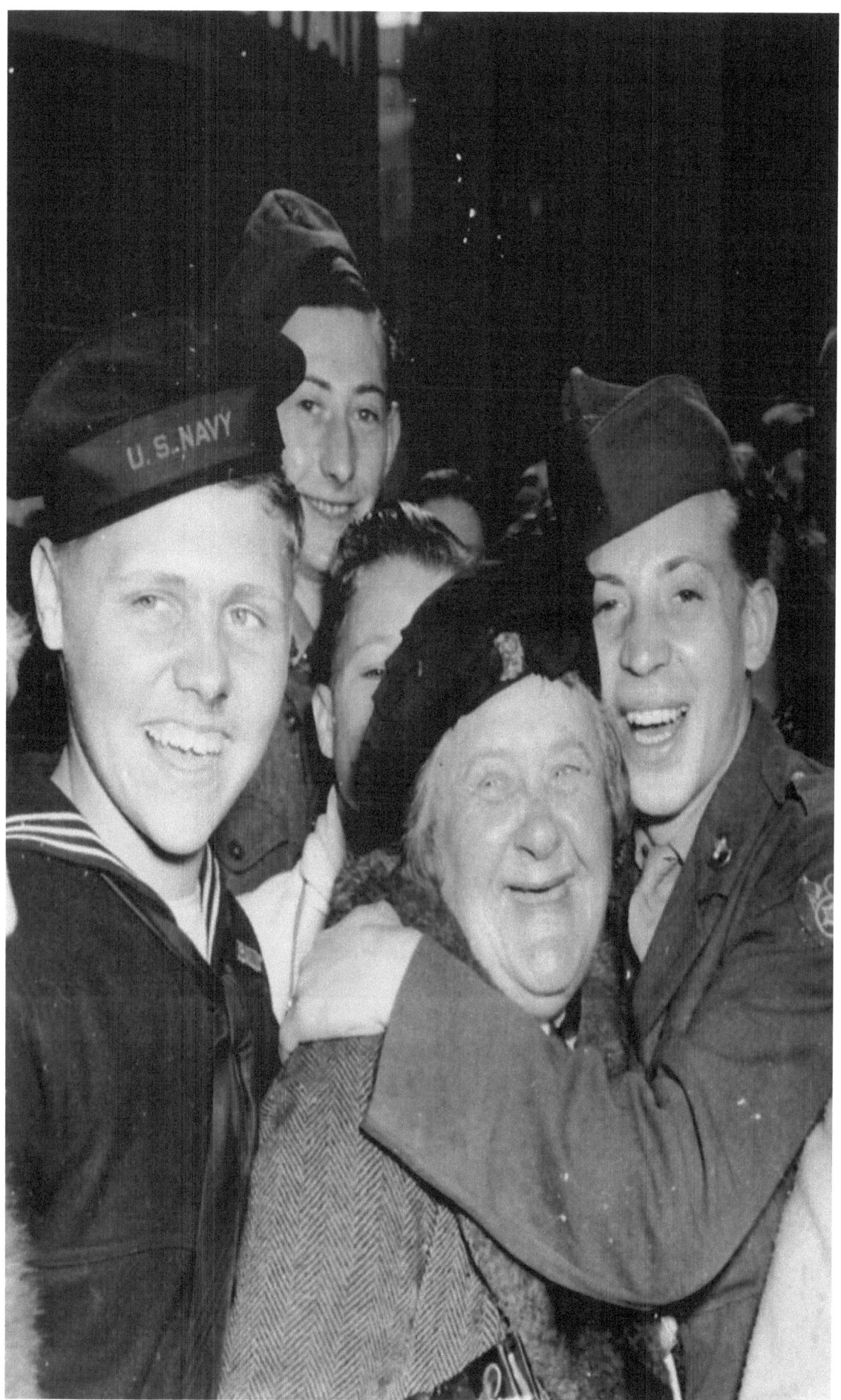

Discussing this image together can encourage memory recall. Give it a try.

Do you remember where you were when you heard the war had ended?

Do you remember the street parties to celebrate the end of the war?

The 8th of May 1945 became forever known as Victory Day. Winston Churchill, King George VI and Queen Elizabeth waved on cheering crowds from the balcony of Buckingham Palace. The future Queen Elizabeth III, then Princess Elizabeth and her sister Princess Margaret were allowed to take part in the street celebrations incognito.

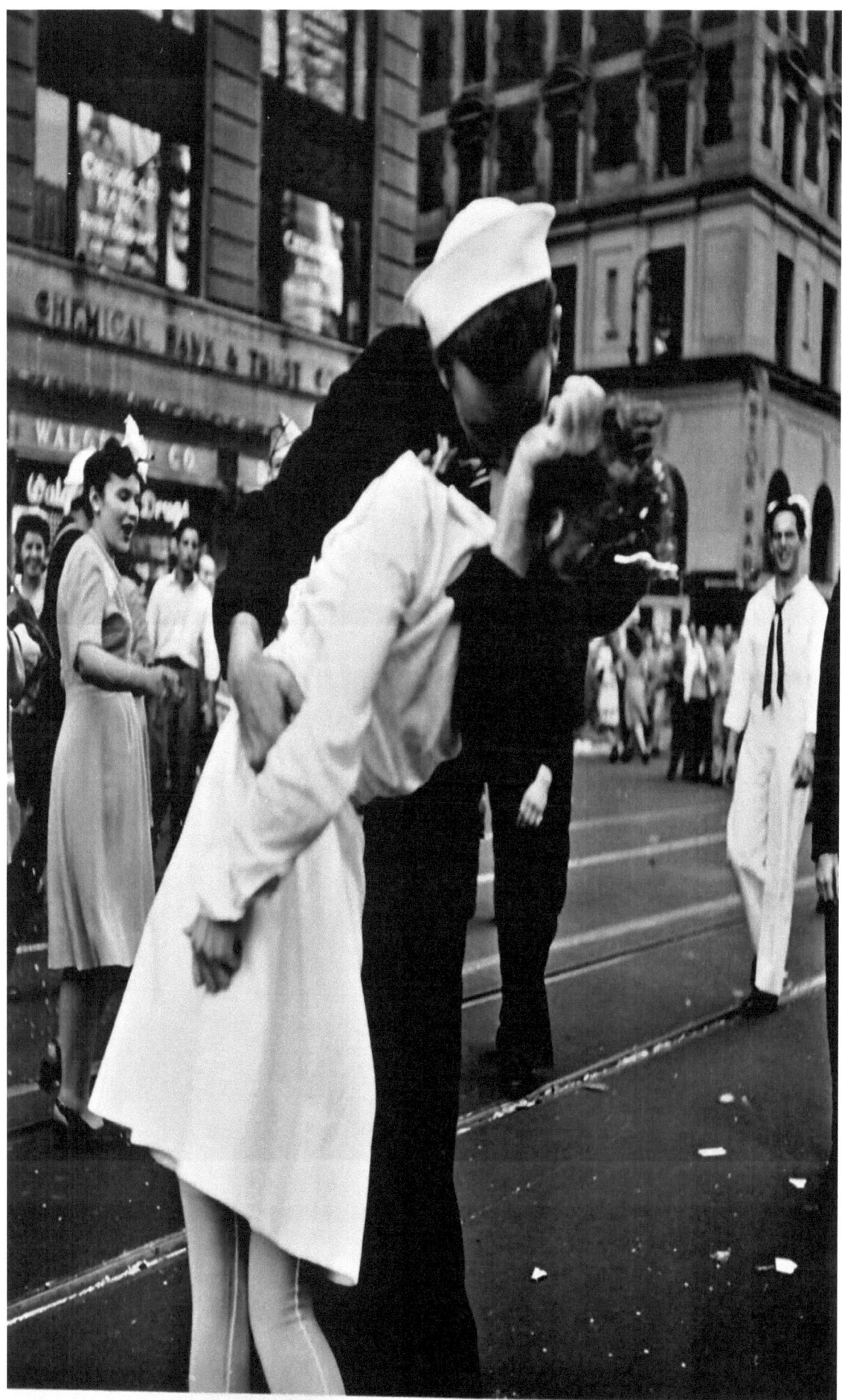

Discussing this image together can encourage memory recall. Give it a try.

Do you remember waiting to hear Winston Churchill announce that the war had ended?

Were you allowed to take part in any of the victory day celebrations?

What did the people who lived beside you do?

Where did everyone go to celebrate that day?

Do you remember any interesting stories from the day?

www.ingramcontent.com/pod-product-compliance
Lightning Source LLC
Chambersburg PA
CBHW050910180526
45159CB00007B/2857